The Renaissance Cycle

*A poetry collection that chronicles overcoming depression
and finding happiness within.*

Christina Anne Hawthorne

I0201109

❧ For Don ☙

*You saved my life once when I didn't think it was worth saving,
and then showed me how to make it grow.
When I needed a path you didn't point,
but instead taught me how to find my way.
I'm still learning, as always I must. You taught me that, too.
Thank you.*

Note

Please remember that I'm not a trained mental health professional, merely someone who's battled the disease all her life. Many environmental factors have worked against me over the years, but I also possess a predisposition. If you're currently suffering depression I urge you to seek help if you haven't done so already. I'll touch on this topic at greater length at the end of the book.

Foreword

This loosely arranged collection's first and shortest part, *Sadness*, examines depression, abuse, heartbreak, loss, tragedy…various sources that have brought me pain over the years. Despite its dark tone I encourage its reading, for it puts what follows in context. The second part, *Awareness*, focuses on opening the mind, discovering truths, and altering perceptions. Part Three, *Reason*, explores choices, mindfulness, determination, and self-reliance. The final part, *Renaissance*, celebrates love, hope, creativity, thankfulness…in general, a happy life.

A table of contents is located near the book's end.

It's my hope you'll find yourself in this collection and, if necessary, seek the road to healing. I suffered the "infinite sadness" for far too long, but assure you *it is* possible to escape that prison and journey to your own Renaissance.

This was my cycle…

Part 1

Sadness

The Infinite Sadness

I'm afraid of something I can't see;
I'm afraid it's inside of me.
Dreams of acceptance and affection,
dreams forever broken.
Forever pain and forever sadness,
forever hopelessness.
Lost in ridicule's twisted sorrow,
lost in no tomorrows.
Save me from this inner darkness;
save me from myself.

Colorless Colors

Grayscale colors in a pre-sun dawn,
life seems that way sometimes…
a fog cloaking your eyes in the morning,
at night easing moisture from your eyes.

Rainbow cheer drawn in black-and-white,
life seems like that sometimes…
arms to hold you that never quite hold you
until you hold yourself and cry.

Springtime blossoms become sticks and stones,
life's like that, too, sometimes…
waiting for someday, day-after-day,
and then waiting becomes wondering and then "why?"

Mind and Heart

So often when I follow my heart I don't know what to do,
for I've often found she has an exceptionally low IQ.
Dancing, frolicking, and living in dreams,
she fails to understand that life is about schemes.

My mind with its logic and reasoning, on the other hand,
always knows how to weigh things and better understand.
Too, it runs the household and manages my heart
only letting her free when writing needs an emotional part.

My heart, she has so much more life she wishes to live
and there's so much love in her that she's yet to give,
but my brain, with its good intentions and justifying
cannot grasp that my aching heart is slowly dying.

Empty Box

My heart has moved on to a place,
a place not found, leaving me—
stranded.
Now, inside my echoing home
I carry the box for my heart—
open-handed.
Where love's gone I do not know,
left me here to wonder—
abandoned.

———

The Call

In that terrible moment your life descends,
sight trapped at the telescope's end.
Vision once possessed becomes distorted,
and what was clear is no longer sorted.

Little noticed is a phone lost through fingers
where strength endowed no longer lingers,
then collapse the knees, muscles unseen,
the falling world stealing your mind, your thinking.

The senses in general are rendered askew
while fumbling for words so suddenly few.
Such is that life-altering moment we fear:
the loss of someone we hold dear.

I See it Now

You don't love me,
I see it now,
so I'll go,
I'll walk away,
before my tears overflow.
Trembling,
shaking,
cursing a life unfair,
I walk away
knowing we were perfect for each other
in every way but one...
I see it now,
you don't love me.

Lines of Time

In silence the lines of time take their toll,
breaking her body, her voice growing thin,
the deathly hollows holding her eyes
little displaying the love within.

Devoted, he walks strong behind her,
his smile masking a hope that's frail,
his spirit willing her to soar
while unseen tears watch her fail.

—◦◦◦—

Never Everlasting

Once, I thought we were something more,
I truly believed we'd walk through that door,
but there'll be no sunrise morning
—not when love became mourning—
not when our future slipped away.

Possibilities dissolved into "unfortunately,"
so much lost prematurely,
the dream, seemingly amaranthine,
became half-a-dream,
a tarnish on the broken heart I've hidden away.

The magic that sparked at the start
became lonely candles in the dark,
and now your cold perfection in our parting
is proof we were never-everlasting,
a final hurt as you turn and walk away.

But It Didn't Have to be that Way

Little girl huddled in the corner, her tears escaping swollen eyes,
fear and misery surrounded her while ignorance spread its lies.

But it didn't have to be that way
through those nights colored gray.
She cried for love, I see that now,
trembling in a room without a home.

Little girl huddled in the corner, her fear masking secret lies,
in a place with no protection, nowhere to hide.

But it didn't have to be that way,
it was black and white, it wasn't gray.
She cried for hope, I see that now,
trembling in a room without a home.

Little girl huddled in the corner seeing through my own eyes,
if I look long enough I still touch the sadness and rationalize.

But it didn't have to be that way,
though my heart escaped the gray.
Faith and strength were hope and love,
trembling in a room without a home.

Evergreen Blue

Scars upon a color rich world
destroying evergreen blue.
Contradictions awaiting explanation,
monotone perceptions ignoring the hues.
The death, not of nature,
but of human kind.
A tragic outcome...
the collective mind running out of time.

Reflective Darkness

Tears in my eyes where fear wears my features,
gazing at the darkness strangling the mirror.

One shaking hand lingers on the reflective side,
but recoils upon seeing what's inside.

Cast me away before it's too late;
thrust me aside before the reflection escapes.

My heart has gone cold and only self-loathing remains.

Remembering the Night

How vivid remains the night.

Sagging clouds illuminated below,
whispering rain catching in the trees,
the leaves bent beneath the teardrop weight
above empty reflections sprayed upon the street.

In the park the grass glistened where the glow allowed,
your storming eyes seemingly not your own,
my eyes tearing before you'd made a sound.

Desperate search for a smile
upon lips cast in frown.
Arms that once held me
held distant and down.

Cruel words stung where rain couldn't go…
I cried, my balance died,
my hearing afire upon rejection.

Shackled in disbelief,
your back adieu,
my lips whispering,
"I loved you…"

Fire

Do you hear the drums, my love,
beating below the thunder?
The city is burning and casting my reason asunder.

On that distant horizon, my love,
is where I see you and I,
walking a road to happiness that's paved with delight.

If you could feel my heart, my love,
you'd know it beats for you,
forever and always a home that is the truth.

I'd have you kiss me once more, my love,
as if the first time came to pass,
but instead there's only longing each night that ever-lasts.

—⁂—

Love & Pain

Excited, I rushed to the door of my emptiness,
for I thought that Love was there on the step,
but he wasn't; he was nowhere to be seen,
he'd taken up living elsewhere, quite happily.

Instead, Pain was at my door, so I invited him in,
bringing only himself and all that he is.
Though he was unkind and cursed me with blame,
I knew cruel nights would comfort just the same.

Now, Pain hits me, especially when I long for Love,
it hurts and I cry, but I won't ask him to leave,
for at least Pain is here for me when I'm alone
because Love came not, he found another home.

I won't be with Pain always, only till the end,
so until then Pain beats me and bruises me bad.
Truly, my Pain will always be here for me
holding me through our long, twisted tragedy.

—⚬⚬⚬—

Dinner for One

I thought of you today
as I prepared my meal…
a can off the shelf.
There were melting candles,
a little something special
while I forced food upon myself.
An empty exercise
to help me feel
the way you made me feel
before you left.

It Survives

A ghastly face behind my eyes
stares from within the solitude inside,
always asking, "why,"
always suspecting lies,
and always the infinite sadness survives.

Desperation screams for love and hides,
but finds only punishment inside.
Always tears are cried,
always torment in my mind,
and always the infinite sadness survives.

I truly thought the day would arrive,
when I'd escape the pain inside.
Always I think, "This time,"
always time dies,
and always the infinite sadness survives.

Part 2

Awareness

The Renaissance Cycle

What You Could See

Days crawled by
holding me in their suffocating embrace,
weeks of lingering pain,
each harrowing like the days.
Months, years,
each plagued with moments of tears—
like the moment I'm having here.

If only I didn't miss you so much,
if only our parting didn't bear sadness.
Could that your eyes find these words
they might discern only anguish,
but please do see,
I'm trying to extract who you saw in me,
I'm trying to believe as you believed.

Just in Time

So many stories,
so many fears.
Shaking, quaking,
year after year.
Childhood memories,
erased from my name.
Fighting, raging,
day after day.
Anger in darkness,
fists clenched tight.
Drinking, screaming,
night after night.
Past turns to present,
my life becomes mine.
Forgiving, healing,
just in time.

Embracing

There are nights when I hold myself tight,
but tight isn't tight enough
when it's my own arms that hold me.

There came a point when I realized
that what I was holding was emptiness,
that part of loneliness no one can see.

Embraced pain was a liar holding my hand
as it drove my knees to find the floor,
covering my lips and their silent pleas.

When my shaking hands dare to extend,
to reach for the hope that faith tells me exists,
that's when I'll find that love is waiting for me.

Here and Not Here

I thought we were together,
but instead we're divided,
accomplished via changed positions
…yours one-sided.

I discovered I was abandoned
though you're still around,
and now I'm left wondering
where your truth can be found?

Your presence isn't enough
…doesn't qualify as devotion.
Sitting there breathing
doesn't qualify as emotion.

❦

Emerging from the Ruins

Waiting.
Waiting for someone to want me for who I am,
not as my past
or my circumstance,
for I'm not those things,
they don't define ME.

Wondering

You ignore me and look the other way,
respond with only a sigh,
leaving me to wonder why,
until I question my understanding.

You say I'm wrong and turn away,
not offering explanation,
nor allowing conversation...
dismissing my words out of hand.

My loneliness is the game you play,
me pondering your meaning,
until I'm wondering,
is my sin having an opinion...?

Contraction

Truth
fading.
Deceit
surrounding.
Compromise
surrendering.
Peace
dying.
Suffering
continues…

Fade Towards the Light

Is there a more divine courage
than continuing the fight
when faced with a body failing
while your mind fades to twilight?

I think not, dear heart.

A sweet whisper to you this night
for your frailty has again shown me
that all that's best in you
is what humanity should strive to be.

Treasuring Time

I've lost so many hours…
shredded paper on my fingers
carried on the breeze.

Too, I've lost days,
days spent languishing in bed
and no longer remembered.

Time long gone,
entire years wasted,
too much lifetime lamented.

Still, there's the future
where time holds possibilities
if I treasure the hours and days.

Cold

Frigid breath,
bitterness,
anger on the breeze.
Glacial glare,
remembrance,
unforgiving freeze.

Dripping lies,
truth for naught,
ire instead of thaw.
Polar words
never sought.
Sincerity?…chilly fraud.

Goodnight

Lights shining bright,
glowing,
ablaze with knowing,
flashing words,
showing pictures also heard,
lashing the gaze,
trying to amaze,
streaking fast
and built to last.
Yet, nature's wonder
steals the thunder.
Human bulbs
sooth and console,
incandescent,
fluorescent,
neon,
halogen,
atomic above the ground—
and then a sound...
When we're gone they're gone
while the sun carries on,
the stars and moon
forgetting our lights all too soon.

Spiral

Hate,
jealousy,
bitterness…
a single drop
and then another,
the more you take
the more they make
for a habit that grows,
reaping the anger sown,
ever-expanding its demands
until the rage can't understand…
eventually it's no longer projected outward,
but instead collects its host.

My Stage

So young I was and on my knees,
broken, despairing, in a Greek tragedy.

Gray moon dusk behind masks in half-light,
whispers cried out wrapped in half-life.

Seeds of pain's theatre sown in my youth,
where lies I was told became the truth.

Despairing I was, trapped on that stage
that became my prison in a different age.

Drafting more misery in that life grown ill,
my poisoned chorus preaching death, until…

In my empty hands my eyes did witness
a means to rebuild and rewrite the illness.

Discarding the mask the sun I did feel,
hope's radiance and applause for real.

I departed fear's stage no longer broken;
hope hadn't died and despair was a lesson.

Trust

It's a test,
in the larger matter of trust:
You can drop your cat
and always it'll land on its feet,
but never will it feel safe in your arms.

This Morning

Waking hazy and confused,
shades of déjà vu.
Thoughts whispered to myself,
a reality screamed in stealth.
Wandering in my wondering,
wondering in my wandering.
Repetitive realization…
again and again and again,
"Today
I'm not the person I was yesterday."

Seeing

Free to be
are you,
are we,
and with it comes
responsibility.
Yet, days pass
and we fail to see
the hurt and pain
inflicted on humanity.
It's in the eyes of those
we pass each week
in public places
we cross silently,
and all the while
we fail to greet,
if only with a smile.
See not the human image,
but instead, the human being inside.

Someone

I can only be myself
and not someone else,
for someone else is for someone else to be.
If I'm not true to my mind
and am hollowed with lies,
then my life is tied to a false self and not to me.

My Crossing Over

In the dark
I saw the sunrise
coming over the ridge,
reminding me I was alive.
I basked in that golden heaven,
crying tears that told me I'd survived.
And with a silent gasp that wasn't my last
I came to realize the radiating light included me.
That instant my frantic struggles concluded
in a place where my heart was set free.
It was there my wandering ended
and I found my walking feet.
Slowing in the moment
I discovered
—me.

Part 3

Reason

The Renaissance Cycle

Past Portraits in the Rain

The more I wonder who I was
the more I realize how I've changed,
and though old faces linger in the fog
each of "me" does eventually fade.

My yesteryears linger outside…
past portraits in the rain.
Falling drops strike faces
losing definition until they're drained.

Other selves bid me goodbye,
melancholy smiles rendered drifting wisps,
and when wrung canvases are gathered
the painful past becomes the mist.

Choice

Fear,
unbridled,
unnecessary,
conjured within my mind
where none should reside,
threatening to spread,
to seize control.

Fight or flight,
for me to choose,
for me to decide.
To stand my ground
where the monster resides
or run away...
I choose to fight.

The Road

Starting over isn't failure,
it isn't retreat,
it's stirring one's soul,
it's renewal,
it's a new branch on life's tree.

Don't surrender your hope
when it's never too late…
this minute,
this second,
embrace hope, don't wait.

This is the road I'm on:
discovering what real life is about.
It's outrunning the fear.
It's embracing the wonder.
It's a mountaintop shout.

Bridge

Maybe I've found the bridge
between where I've been
and where I'm going.
Maybe it was beneath my feet
all along.
My thanks to each and every one of you
who placed a stone.

Looking Back

I've traveled far,
narrowly missed catastrophe,
crossed rivers and mountains
and the miles in-between.
Yet, as I stand upon the brink
and look back upon my journey
I realize the most important steps
were the ones that led to me.

Mercy

Behind your scowl,
where the inner demons played with your soul,
I'd sometimes glimpse the man I admired
and who made me proud.

But the demons won,
twisting your soul until your pain was mine,
taking away the father who could have been
until it was as if you'd died.

I ran away once
and in the running saved the future I'd thought not to have,
discovered the good you shared before the dark days,
before your collapse.

Now your light dims
and this broken heart that finally forgave and tried to forget
whispers in the back of my mind that it's time…
have mercy or regret.

Between Before and After

Escaping my cloudy past,
leaving my rearview perceptions afar,
and favoring the solid ground
that exists between before and after…

At first screaming,
thrashing,
and twisting in fear
until I realized
my feet had settled
upon the balance I hold dear.

Ahead,
my life stretching outward,
—boundless muse—
and yet
there's only one direction:
the direction I choose.

In an Instant

So many rationalizations over time...

In an instant your words told me all I needed to know.
In an instant I glimpsed beyond the façade.
In an instant I finally saw the truth.

You've no respect for the person before you,
you've no respect for me.
That long moment standing there
became eternity as love became fleeting.
Comprehension spread to my heart
as I walked away, seething.
At the corridor's end I turned a corner
on my way to self-esteem.

I Believe

I believe
my life has endured,
has waited
for that special someone.
I believe
my heart has awakened,
has expanded,
with room for two.
I believe
my soul has healed,
has renewed,
to help another.
I believe
purpose has emerged,
has materialized,
to show me the way.
I believe
I believe in me.

Procrastination

Waiting for the right time,
waiting for the planets to align.
Waiting, waiting, waiting…
procrastination does nothing,
yet works hard to keep me at bay.

Again I languish and linger,
again I squander and it gloats.
Again and again and again…
until I grab delay by the throat,
look it in the eye, and toss it outside.

Mourning After

The morning after I died
I held your hand to help you understand.
I kissed your cheek while you slept in my arms
and watched your steps to keep you from harm.
My energy allows me to not fade away
because its source is the love you share each day.

Frequency

Four walls stared back for too long
while I searched the emptiness within sight.
Long believing myself undeserving
while my heart bled and I cried through the night.

An intrepid adventurer I've recently become
and rendered the darkness benign,
not cursing gloom or burying happiness,
but appreciating the contrasts assigned.

Existing in harmony establishes my balance
and frees the gift within me.
I'm but one vibration in this vast universe
who's finally found her frequency.

Human Choice

The sun is bright.
That means it's doing right.
The sky is blue.
That's what it's supposed to do.
The rain is falling,
for that's its calling.
What am I supposed to do?
Anything I choose.

The Other Side

There was no bargain,
no pact made face-to-face,
you've discovered the other side
and they think you've lost your way.

Still, you'll move on,
yes, there comes that time,
and so you don't look back
when you reach the other side.

Self-actualization
elicits a brief hollow
when you reach the other side
and know they won't follow.

Seeing Me

A crowded mind, wispy clouds lacking substance,
a plaything with no soul...
Is that how you see me?
Please tell me, "No."

Dispensable emotions of no consequence,
tears and smiles only for show...
Is that how you see me?
Please tell me, "No."

A useful thing for handling without conscience,
soon inconvenient, soon disposed...
Is that how you see me?
Please tell me, "No."

Heart and mind, body and soul, a unique essence,
requiring respect...
That's how I see me.
That's what I expect.

Dear Humanity

I sometimes wonder
what the world would be
if we all did our best,
if we settled for no less,
if we, the human race,
moved forward together.
Perhaps it can't be,
perhaps the cynics are right
and hatred is our destiny,
but either we're moving ahead side-by-side
or we're stepping off the cliff in single file.
And so I keep wondering...

Pathways

Worry and guilt lead to confusion,
the pathways in our minds running amuck,
a spider's web created while drunk.

I see now that opening my mind
isn't about complexity,
but rather, simplicity.

Simplicity is what understanding inspires
rather then chaos,
rather then what leads the mind to "lost."

The Girl Who Never Lived

I've awoken, for the past is over
and long since done.
New days await a new light
where there's sun.

My prison, my seclusion,
I knew it well.
I set each brick to secure my isolation,
my personal hell.

To there I escaped inner torment,
unrelenting abuse.
To there I fled,
my rope a custom noose.

Now, outside that shattered prison
looking in,
I shed a tear for the girl who cowered,
never lived.

Weep not for a youth gone by,
my dear sad one,
you can smile within the me I am now
beneath the sun.

Setting Myself Free

I see the truth in the sunrise,
in its hopeful aspect.
I feel the truth in my heart,
in the dreams it protects.

Dreams die hard,
my determination harder still.
I'll overcome the challenges
because I have the will.

No time like the present,
no time like now.
Don't know how I'll do it,
but I'll do it somehow.

Transition

I returned to where once there was a beginning
only to find an end.
Ashes to ashes,
the past did descend.
I walked away, gentle hands supporting
a heart on the mend.
Before my eyes
the clouds did part and the future ascend.

Time and Timelessness

Looking back at yesterdays
I see hazy goals and wishful things,
yearning, then enduring
life's trials and confusion.

As for tomorrows,
of vivid dreams and aspirations,
I'll sprint towards opportunity
with eyes and arms wide open.

But for now and today,
between time and timelessness,
my heart's desires shall prevail
when riding the thankful winds.

Part 4

Renaissance

The Renaissance Cycle

Passion

I'm ready,
ready to jump the fence,
ready to race towards the sun
unbridled,
unbroken.
You'd better tie my passion down
or I'll be gone,
running where I want,
where I'm appreciated,
unrestrained,
unreserved.
Can't wait to let this passion burn
in the sweltering night
where there's no corral to contain,
just me embracing the open field
unapologetic,
unrelenting,
and unwilling to tie this passion down.

The Beckoning

Somewhere beyond,
past the meadow where the forest begins to grow,
where the mountains start to rise,
came a whispering voice that beckoned,
"Come this way, dear one
who's long been gone,
lost where the tangled vines grow too long.
Venture forth and capture your soul,
become whole—for the first time."
The great weight at the center of who I am
plunged to nevermore,
easing the pain that was the past long gone
and rendering my trembling hands a calming storm.
Dear heart,
the peaceful whispers I hear
must be you guiding me,
for my feet can no longer find the floor when I walk.
This must be what others call "tears of joy,"
this must be me finding happiness.

Teller of Tales

I wish to journey with a teller of tales in a dreamer's dream
following a ferocious lion along a cascading stream...
unicorns frolicking beneath bright crescent bows,
stone towers that ensnare the distant unknown,
my teller of tales forever holding tight my hand and heart.

Mystics, magicians, sorcerers, and wizards all abound;
my love shall speak of them in each cavern, tavern, and town.
Be it deep vale, dense forest, or towering heights,
when together, my love, there'll be such magical nights.
Forever my teller of tales holding me tight and stealing my heart.

✝ ❦ ✝

Insight

There between the misty glow
and the apple blossoms in sunshine
I found understanding,
not profound wisdom
as would be told to all,
but, instead,
my heartbeat's call.
And so I go,
not far away,
yet no longer here,
for though I've sought to touch the sky
and found it beyond my reach
I've learned that the beauty that is this universe
exists deep inside of me.

My Rainy Night

Shivering within my coat,
shimmer and glisten pierce the haze.
Beneath a streetlight
whispered rain falls in waves,
dancing crystal on a pavement palette…
I hold tight my umbrella.

Patter above my head, patter about my feet.

Wrapped in strong embrace,
our bodies chasing away ebony chill.
Breath seeks the fog
summoning a dance wrapped in ethereal
as moisture collects on warming skin…
I relish the heat.

Droplets ripple and spread, droplets ripple and flee.

His dark eyes caress my face,
happiness warming the tears in my eyes.
I cannot look away,
my gaze following the fingertip upon my smile,
and his beckoning me.
My lips meet his.

Cat Tale

My kitty,
she's itchy
in her own fur.
Took a brush,
made her lush,
and now she purrs.
Meow.

❧❧❧

As if Out of a Dream

Angels, embodied in everyday people,
to whom I'm thankful.
Kindness blooming in my garden,
and it's delightful.
Hands that grasp with love's touch,
and my heart is grateful.
Salvation, it seems, is as if out of a dream,
but in reality tangible.

Morning Cup

Still sleepy, but—
there's always a "but"
and it's time to wake.
Open heavy eyes…
Sigh…stretch.
Kitty eyes looking at me.
That's no surprise.
Sigh…stretch again,
slide off the bed…
stand, stumble, and wobble.
Starting the coffee…
Feed hungry felines.
Pills in me…one, two, three.
Sigh, yeah, way too many.
Coffee aroma…oh, yes…
Cup in my hand,
sugar, cream, stir, sip, and sigh again,
but heavier this time.
A horrific scream close by…
ah, it's just the caffeine bidding me "good morning."
Oh my, oh wow, oh yeah, oh how I'm ready, don't ya know.
Yeah, I've got things to do, people to see, places to go…
what a glorious day this is going to be!

This Writer's Mind

Breath of my soul
drawn through my pen
casts forth my thoughts,
upon each page is it spread.
All eyes shall see
my need,
my disease,
and the cure that sets me free.
Open your mind and I'll share the remedy…

Spidey, Ya Got No Righty

Spiders,
one left, two left, three left, four,
and on the other side they've got four more.
Yes, all those legs and too many eyes to mention
leaving me quite unsure of their intentions.
Watching me,
chasing me,
and always using my superior size to their advantage.
Ah, that tangled web they weave
and it's always in places I can't believe.
Yikes, the very thought of spiders nearly kills me dead,
my arachnophobia is so bad
I'd have to use a picture of a puppy instead.

In Your Sleep

Rest your weary eyes, my dearest one,
discover the slumber possessing your fantasy.
In darkness I'll whisper words in your ear
and tempt your thoughts towards ecstasy.
My caress will guide you to the dawn
where I await you on the far side of your dreams.

My List

A thin, full dress,
just enough for the breeze to play with
on a sunny day in Paris…
that's on my list.

Where the sun comes first,
ocean waves to shore's first kiss
below my coastal perch…
that's on my list.

A soft, cozy night,
the fire inside, outside the mist
far away eyes alight…
that's on my list.

An endless highway,
sunrise to sunset in loving bliss
while the music plays…
that's on my list.

Realizing dreams and schemes,
no details missed,
and sharing it with all of you…
that's on my list.

Cat Hair

Dear kitty,
your hair up to there,
up my nose,
and on my chair;
adrift, ceiling high,
scattered low,
and in my eye.
To everything I make
it's clinging,
including the cake.
Amidst it all you're so smug,
cleaning your toes
and coating the rug.

❧❦❧

Together

You're my counterweight,
my balance,
the harmony that soothes my soul.
Come to me, my love…
love me,
and together we'll ignite the cold.

Christmas Wish

He for whom the day is named
is the tie upon the gift that's giving,
for the gifts we give
are meant for all among the living.
Let us sing in a voice that is one,
shared in thankfulness and rejoicing,
spread one heart to another,
hand-in-hand, and all embracing.

Youthfulness Everlasting

Aged hand,
a century passed beneath your fingertips,
but hasn't stolen the smile upon your lips.
I look to the wall,
to the pictures whispering there,
to the happiness the monochrome lays bare.
Touching a finger to the frame
I come to realize
that joy is in more than the eyes.
The happiness within
is carried forward on the inside
where there's no reason for it to ever die.
Now I have tears of joy,
a youthfulness everlasting,
the thankfulness never ending.

What I Am

I am fire,
I am smoke,
I'm the renewal coming behind.
I am dusk,
I am dawn,
I'm weaving a thin, gray line.
I am darkness,
I am light,
I'm the solar eclipse in the sky.
I am life,
I am death,
I'm existing between times.
I am thoughts,
I am words,
I'm creativity and one of a kind.

Before Everlast Descended

How fortunate I am
that in that life-defining moment
I opened my eyes before everlast descended.

I hesitated where others succeeded
and upon opening my eyes I realized,
we don't lose hope—we lose the ability to see it.

Before it's too late
open your senses to see what you've lost,
that's hope,
and in the instant following there's thankfulness.
Savor it too.

Writing Fantasy

Deep within me…
a flame for a candle,
a word upon the page,
a world unlike another,
and magic for a mage.

Deep within me…
I flicker no more,
I escape this shell,
I transcend the dream
casting an all-consuming spell.

The Chaos in Me

Sometimes
when I look inside
my own mind
I see
more mystery
than clarity:
right brain,
left brain,
struggling for sane;
a writer's store
of fantasy lore
where less is more.
Don't get me wrong,
for like a song
the harmony is strong,
and the truth is,
in this life I live
I've much to give,
for the chaos in me
is thankfully
creativity.

Paws

There ought to be a law
against clever paws with claws
coming from up high,
down low,
and even behind.
There's no safe haven from paws
snagging,
scratching,
and generally snatching
whatever they can grab
or nab
before they run away.
Alas, I lament
that skirt,
that top,
and those pants,
for they were gorgeous
when they came through the door,
but not anymore.

❧❧

A Writer's Wish

Joy of wonder, fill this writer's sight anew
and glisten child-like eyes with the morning's dew.
Please summon inspiration and chronicle a hero's quest
to where starlight night bathes a silver shadow's rest.

Upon my plunge into imagination's vivid abyss
I'll lose myself in passion's peak and each lover's kiss.
For evermore I'll scrawl where before there was no trace
until I sprawl in a golden meadow deep in sleep's embrace.

Mindful Paths

There's an intersection
where the paths in my mind meet,
one of many, many to see.
The paths that serve me
prosper in perpetuity,
all forever, forever for me.
Those I find harmful
fade to transparency,
into disuse, for they don't deserve me.

Melting

Words escape me now,
now that you're close, looking my way.
My breath stills, the room melts,
and all else fades away.

Our eyes in silent dance,
no words while the band plays on.
My fever heats, the drums beat...
all resistance gone.

Must breath or pass away,
no one else effects me like this.
My trembling, wanting, needing,
your lips, our kiss.

Where There's Hope

Within the dreams that nourish
lies the truth of our existence,
inspiration for the ages
to sustain hours cast darkest.
When illness plagues your heart
and from your eyes flows unimpeded, too,
I'll lift that which makes humanity great
and offer that love to you.

❧

My Champion

Lay not your sword at my feet, my love,
upon bended knee do not rest.
My heart you captured long ago…
my love has not passed.

Dragons have bowed before you,
carried you across plains and seas
to distant, mystic lands
such as my eyes have never seen.

Upon unicorns have you journeyed
to dells, the elves and their trees,
a wooded mystery world
wrapped as tales and presented to me.

I've seen your fire and felt your touch,
my dearest traveling one,
so please take this sword I do now hold…
it's a kiss I desire, my love.

†❤†

Oft Told Tale

The tale of my existence is an oft told tale
spoken not on chilled evenings beneath a listening moon,
nor uttered when contrasts swath the afternoon.

Instead, it dwells in a quiet soul's creative solitude,
often silent, forever awaiting this heart's desire to share
feathered explanations here before they're somewhere.

See me now: laughter breaking upon nothing for sure,
a winsome candle clinging to the flame's fleeting glow,
fingers polishing magic on a forgotten realm's sorrow.

Hush the frantic winds beseeching my demise,
gather elusive kindling burning when my heart is tight,
and perhaps I'll whisper an oft told tale beneath desire's night.

My Renaissance

A note of hope I hold,
wrapped in passion's light,
read beneath a writer's moon,
in a silver meadow's night.

My aforementioned hope,
penned in revelation's ink,
is a creative flowering
more extensive than you'd think.

This is my renaissance,
where all bestowed gifts do merge,
where I find my center,
where thankfulness is given birth.

Afterword

These poems, written over a 3-year period, contain the experiences and emotions accumulated over a lifetime. In fact, parts of *The Infinite Sadness* and *It Survives* are derived from poems I wrote as a teen.

This project came about after several dear people suggested I compile my poetry and publish it. Given that I think of myself as a fiction writer first I was flattered and deeply honored they'd make such a request. Time passed, I grew a little, more wounds healed, and finally the thought entered my mind, *Why not?*

And then a strange thing happened.

What began as a favor became a passion. I don't consider myself a poet in the classic sense, but sensed that my words might allow others to see it's possible to recover happiness.

I'd amassed over 450 poems, some awful, and realized I faced a daunting task. For six months I sifted through poetic musings and memories, but eventually I discovered those most near and dear to my heart. Those 87 poems were then separated into four parts.

This project wasn't about reaching the end of a journey, for in growing there is no end, but instead was about achieving sufficient peace and self-actualization to allow me to discover the happiness within.

The Renaissance Cycle

An Urgent Message

If your life is such that you're suffering depression or anxiety then I urge you to seek help immediately. Friends, family members, counselors, doctors, clergy, hot lines…the resources these days are numerous. Call someone. Make contact with another human being. Talk.

"We don't lose hope—we lose the ability to see it."

Depression reassures us with whispers urging isolation. It steals our reason, awareness, and sight while goading us to cut ourselves off from help.

I know. Believe me, I know.

More than once I stood at the edge of the abyss, the worst moment coming the day before I decided to find help. Eventually, too, I found the right fit for me, I found the man who saved my life. Now, here I am 9 years later writing about it. Even so, after half a lifetime of depression I realized remaining healthy must be a lifelong effort. For me that meant not relying on drugs, which my body little tolerates.

Depression becomes a habit, not because we're weak, but because "short-cut" pathways are created in the brain like with any repetitive task. Thus, with each occurrence it becomes easier for it to happen again.

So, I'll say it again, seek help. Seeking help is a sign of taking charge, a sign of strength.

Please, do it.

Part 1 Contents: *Sadness*

Part 2 Contents: *Awareness*

Part 3 Contents: *Reason*

Part 4 Contents: *Renaissance*

Acknowledgements

Poetry is a more solitary pursuit, but those who've encouraged mine are great in number. I'd be amiss if I didn't mention my daughters and everyone who's ever provided an inspiring word. Those words helped more than you know. Too, a special "thank you" to my sister who gave me a blank book and told me to "keep writing" exactly 38 years ago. This collection has been a long time coming and is a dream come true.

Biography

Christina Anne Hawthorne, originally from the US east coast, now resides in the breathtaking western Montana mountains with her two cats. Frequent walks serve as vital exercise and continual inspiration. Her longtime fascination with the fantasy genre led to her reimagining it and creating the world of Ontyre. Currently, on her new website is the free online serial, *Last Word Before Dying*. This autumn she'll publish a more ambitious tale, *Where Light Devours*, that also takes place in that world.

Connections:

Website:	http://christinaannehawthorne.com
Blog:	http://christinahawthorne.wordpress.com
Facebook:	www.facebook.com/ChristinaAnneHawthorne
Twitter:	https://twitter.com/CA_Hawthorne
Pinterest:	http://pinterest.com/christinahawtho

www.ingramcontent.com/pod-product-compliance
Lightning Source LLC
Chambersburg PA
CBHW021134020426
42331CB00005B/762